HOPE

May 2017

TBI Advocacy & Education
HOPE
MAGAZINE
*"Supporting the
Brain Injury Community"*

Welcome

TBI HOPE MAGAZINE

Serving All Impacted by Brain Injury

May 2017

Publisher
David A. Grant

Editor
Sarah Grant

Contributing Writers
Nicole Bingaman
Lethan Candlish
Darron Eastwell
Donna O'Donnell Figurski
Barb George
Natalie Griffith
Lori Harrison
Ralph Poland
Melissa Robison

Amazing Cartoonist
Patrick Brigham

*FREE subscriptions at
www.TBIHopeMagazine.com*

Welcome to the May 2017 issue of TBI HOPE Magazine!

The May issue of TBI HOPE Magazine marks the 26th issue of our publication, something my wife Sarah and I are immensely grateful to be a part of.

Over the last several years, we have been able to bring you stories of inspiration from around the globe. While most of the commonly cited brain injury facts are based on US statistics, brain injury knows no boundaries.

Last month, I was able to present at the Brain Injury Canada semi-annual conference at Saint John, New Brunswick. Speaking with local survivors at the conference was the high point of our trip. Brain injury does not discriminate based on age, gender, or address, and affects people worldwide.

This month's issue features stories by survivors, caregivers & family members. *The Day I Broke My Brain* by Australian Darron Eastwell is a reminder that brain injury can happen anywhere.

As always, I welcome your feedback. Please feel free to email me directly at david@tbihopeandinspiration.com.

Peace,

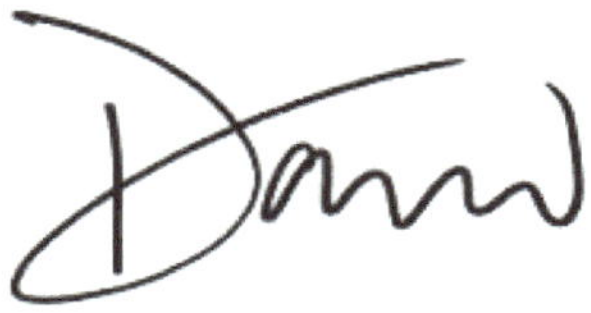

David A. Grant
Publisher

Contents

Over 5.3 Million People Live Daily with a Brain Injury

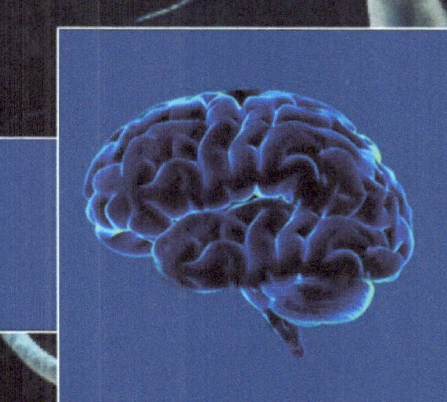

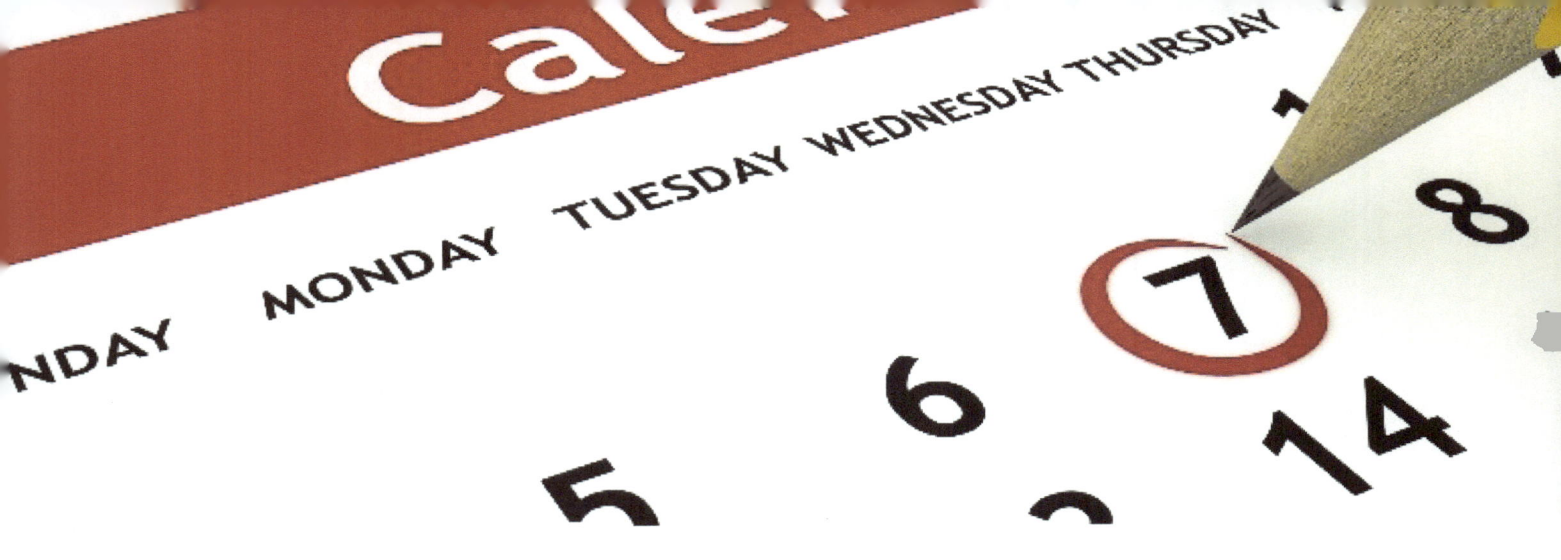

1825 Days

By Lori Harrison

One thousand, eight hundred and twenty-five days is how long it's been since I got my injury. On that sunny day, I never thought that walking back into the grocery store would change my whole life and the old me would die and the new me would survive.

No, I wasn't shot or stabbed. I walked into the grocery store and didn't see a massive puddle of clear liquid laundry soap someone had spilled on the floor. I slid forward and hit my forehead on a shelf. After that, I think I fell backward and cracked my head open. I don't remember falling, but I remember the feeling of sliding toward the shelf and fearing I would hit my head on it. I heard the sound of my head hitting the concrete and then black empty nothingness took me over.

I don't remember a lot about the fall, but after waking up and being unable to move, I felt like a huge lump of coal on the floor. I was soaking wet and thinking I had wet myself, but it turned out to be liquid laundry soap. Someone had spilled the biggest container of laundry soap you could ever think of all over the floor and I was lying in it.

At the time, I wasn't aware that 1825 days later I would still be injured. I didn't think I would have migraine headaches and constant low-level headaches, dizziness, aphasia, problems walking, problems with balance, brain fog, problems with my vision, and problems with light and sound sensitivity on a daily basis. I didn't think 1825 days later I would have sleep problems, high blood pressure, and thyroid problems. All of the symptoms came to me by hitting my head twice.

I'm grateful though. I'm grateful that I lived. I now live in the here-and-now, and in the moment. I am grateful that I have learned how to walk again. I'm still learning. It has taught me patience, which I had very little of, prior to my accident. It has taught me strength - we are a lot stronger than we realize we are! I've had a lot of strife in my life but nothing has tested me as much as this injury.

Today, I have acceptance. It took me three-and-a-half years and many hours of counseling to accept the new me. I truly believe that it's been the hardest part of this journey. Life is truly a journey, not a destination. When we were young, we grew into somebody different as teenagers than who we are as adults. We meet people, we pick up their good and bad habits, and we change. Have I changed with this injury!

Accepting an injury, especially a brain injury, is difficult. It is the hardest thing I've ever done in my life, and if you told me 1500 days ago that I would be able to accept my new life and "The New Me," I would've told you that you were crazy.

"The New Me" is very different than the old me. She's a completely different person with a different personality, with a different outlook on life and a different size and shape. The face that looks back at me in the mirror, the eyes, nose, mouth and ears are the same, but the person who looks back at me is completely different. This person is not one I grew into or developed over time, but one who appeared when my head hit the concrete floor. Today, I accept that.

March 25, 2012, is my new birthday. It's my other birthday and I celebrate every year. The first two years I cried and was so sad. This year I am celebrating. I'm celebrating how far I've come and how much good has come from this injury. I'm planning my favourite seafood dinner for that night for myself, to honour just how strong I really am. I'm also celebrating how lucky I am to belong to a club of brain injury survivors, which I would never have voluntarily joined. We survived and now we are thriving as survivors, different and better than ever.

Meet Lori Harrison

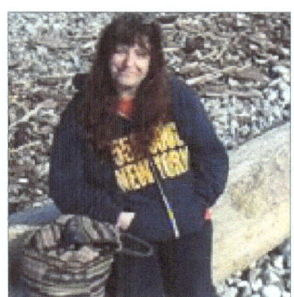

Lori is an essayist and horsewoman having ridden both English and Western. She is hoping to get back in the saddle next year. She is currently on disability and working hard on her recovery. She is getting back to her writing and moving towards being a life coach and advocate for adults, children, and families with TBI or anxiety and depression.

Great works are performed not by strength but by perseverance.

~Samuel Johnson

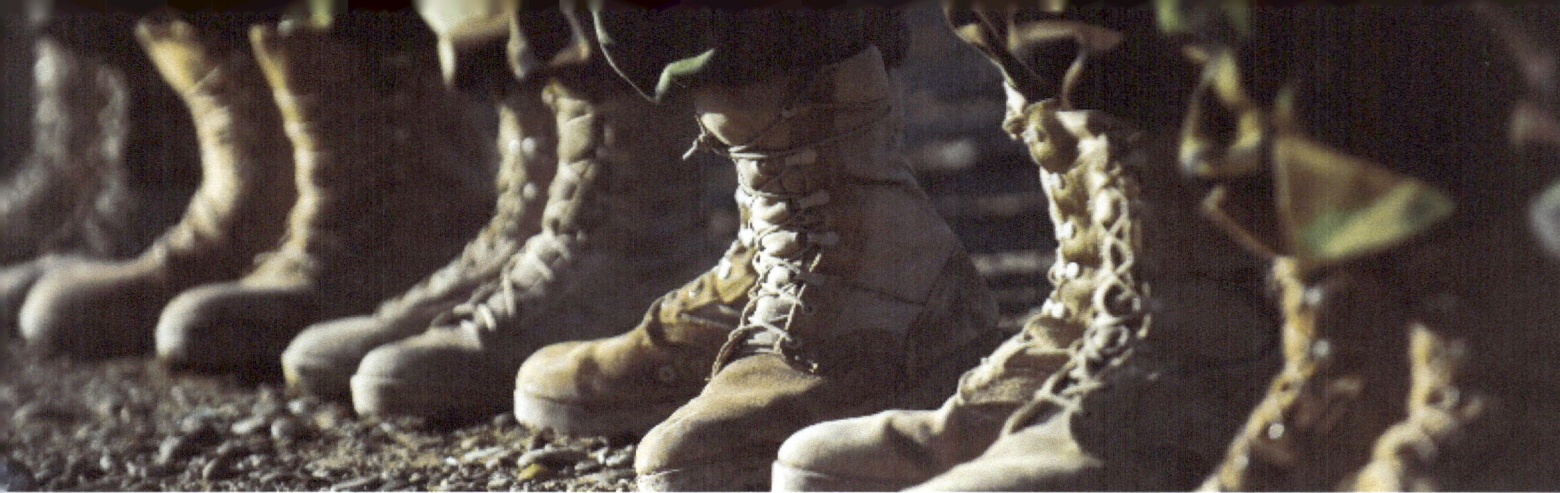

The Fall that Changed it All

By Melissa Robison

I was probably the first soldier in history to volunteer to go to Hot Box training. Under constant simulated attack, with no sleep, little time to eat, and no outside contact aside from my few teammates, yeah it sounded fun to me. It probably was more about me feeling like I had something to prove to the men in my unit, which definitely seemed to be a common theme with me. With very little water and dressed in big, heavy, chemical warfare gear during the summer in Tennessee, I'm sure I was pretty dehydrated when, five days in, I got yanked to go to Air Assault School.

When I first heard about Air Assault School, I had this romanticized vision in my head. I was told it was the most rigorous school a female soldier could get sent to in the Army. Though I was not even done with my specialized training, I put in the orders to go and that was the reason I was stationed in the 101st Airborne Division. I wanted to push myself and the boundaries. I had joined the Army during the first year of coed basic training and was in a field newly opened to females. So, pretty much everything I set out to do was to push the envelope. I grew up having a very tough single mother who rode Fat Boy Harley's, and I was a bit of a tomboy, so basically nothing scared me. I was such a thrill seeker back then, and hell, I still am.

Most people train and rest before the first morning of Air Assault School, where you have to pass a four-mile run and insane obstacle course to get accepted. I, on the other hand, was just glad I had a shower first. Near the end of the first day and course, I passed out at the top of an obstacle called "The Tough One," which was 30 feet tall. I fainted at the top, they said. I was also told that because I didn't have any rope burns on my hands (which would have indicated muscle failure and slid down the rope,) that I just blacked out from fatigue.

The last thing I remember is trying to pull myself over the top beam about three stories up. I woke up surrounded by medics standing over me. Since I was a female and probably slower than all the guys, I'm

Meet Melissa Robison

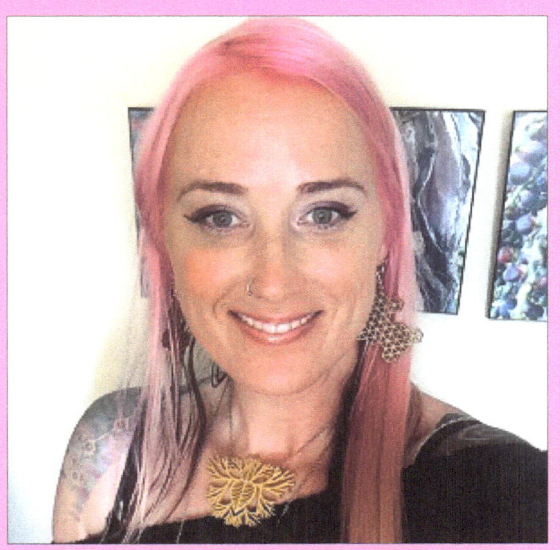

Melissa holds a Bachelor's In Accounting and Master's Degree in Technology Management, she is a recipient of the Massachusetts Women in Public Higher Education Award, and a featured Student of the Week at Bridgewater State University.

A Ttraumatic Brain Injury and PTSD Survivor, Melissa continues to give compassionately though she has debilitating daily health conditions. Melissa served as a member of a highly respected Spiritual Group in Massachusetts, where she volunteered Medium and Healing services.

Melissa believes she chose this difficult path on this Earth, because she is a server to all of humanity, and will always continue to bring light to those needing it most.

guessing I was near the end of the group. There is no instructor positioned at the beginning of an obstacle to tell you how to navigate and pass each obstacle. There is only one instructor at the end to tell you if you passed correctly and flag you to go on to the next.

So, it may have been some time before I was noticed, and I don't know how far an ambulance would have had to come from, or how long the EMT's were standing over me.

I'm guessing I was probably unconscious for 15-20 minutes at least, but no one is sure. Lots of Traumatic Brain Injury (TBI) survivors have a hard time judging how long they were knocked unconscious.

I've been told that it was a good thing I was unconscious for the fall because if I hadn't gone limp I would've broken my back and more. I landed on a hay bail. Apparently, the Army has a better cushion for falls now, haha.

Someone asked me today if I would do it all again, and I instantly said no. I realized yesterday that I have lived the last nineteen years with TBI and PTSD. That is half of my life. With more thoughtful consideration of the question, I honestly would have to say I would not change any of it. My life has been exactly what it was supposed to be.

Yes, I have huge health problems and spend each day wishing I was out hiking again, however, I know there is more in store for me in this life.

I look back and am unable to imagine not having adversity to face. Without these struggles, I wouldn't have to fight so hard to accomplish things and reach my goals; that's what builds character - character I would not trade for one second of a pain-free day, hands down.

COMING IN JUNE 2017

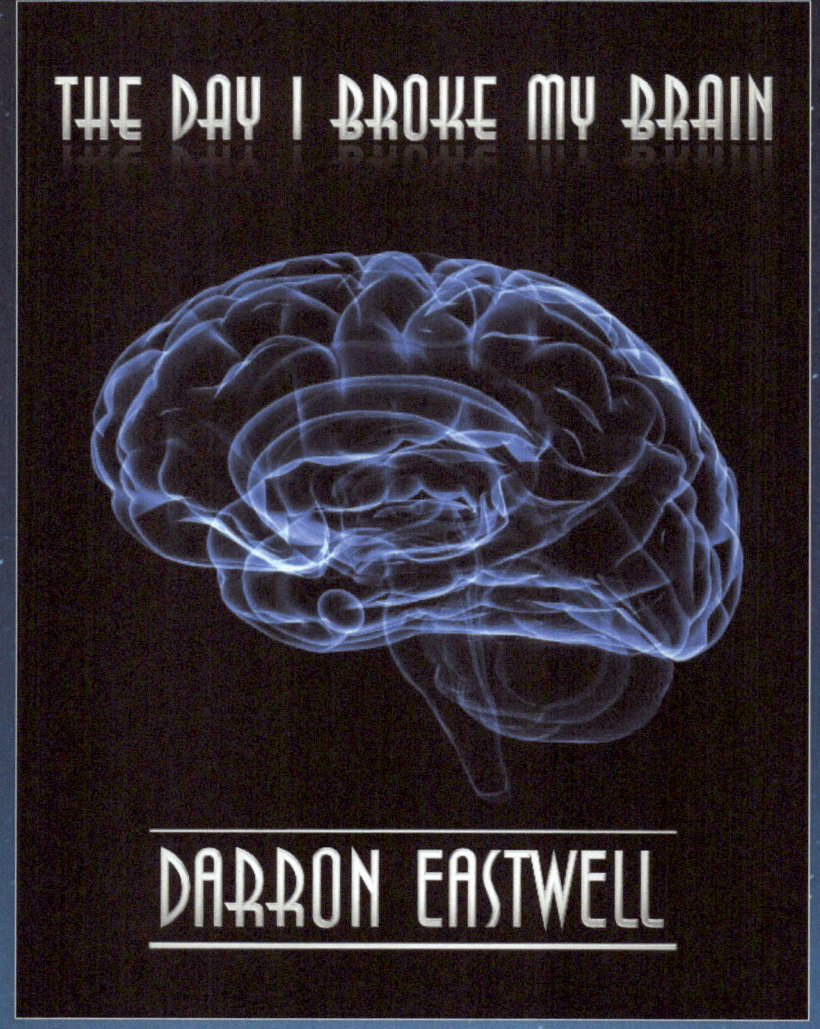

AN INSPIRATIONAL NEW BOOK BY SURVIVOR

DARRON EASTWELL

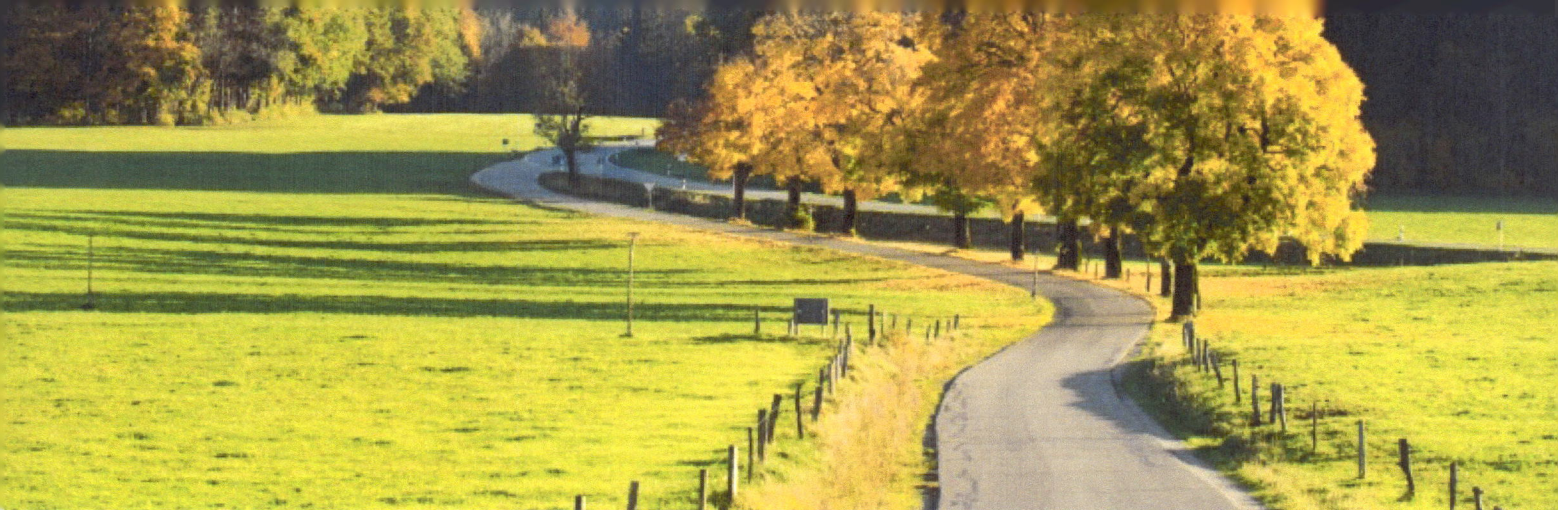

The Gift of My Recovery

By Lethan Candlish

It was early in my senior year of high school when I was called upon to take my sister to her small, rural elementary school for an overnight party as part of the newly established middle school - at the time, there were only four middle-schoolers enrolled. I was a relatively new driver and had just had an adolescent spat with my mother, so it was exciting to get out of the house and just drive.

At the school, after letting my sister run off with her friends, I had a discussion with her middle-school advisor, Eleanor - also my former French teacher. I remember feeling a sense of maturity talking with Eleanor - now I was an almost-adult (17 years old), not just a kid like my sister and her friends, and we could speak about my plans for college and the projects I was involved with. The way she respected my plans while sharing her experiences and the fact that my parents were nowhere near me made it feel like one of my first truly "adult" conversations.

My last memory…I watched my former French teacher wave goodbye, through my rearview mirror, as I drove off into the night.

The accident occurred on a quiet, narrow, country road - it's not the main road between my house and my sister's school, but it's a route that takes a little less time and is much more interesting, especially for a new driver. I don't remember the drive leading up to the accident, but I have been told that a car had just passed me traveling the opposite direction when he saw me lose control (through his rearview mirror) and crash into a telephone pole. My guess is that I was driving a little too fast (10ish miles over the speed limit) and, being relatively new to the road, when I passed the other driver I swerved just enough that my wheel dipped over the side of the narrow, country road, making me lose control for just a moment, but a moment that sent me into the telephone pole. That's my guess at what happened, but it makes sense to me.

What has been documented are the events that followed: the man who witnessed my accident rushed to the nearest farmhouse and banged on the door and asked to use their telephone (this occurred in the BC era - Before Cellphones); fortunately, there had been no other major accidents in the region, so the hospital was able to immediately send their emergency rescue helicopter; the volunteer emergency crew which just happened to include my family's auto-mechanic and friend responded in record time and flew me to Geisinger Medical Center, the large regional hospital; there, I began my journey of recovery.

These are the facts surrounding my accident and rescue - such a textbook-perfect rescue situation that several of my friends have commented on how lucky I was - except that I had an accident. I recognize this relative good fortune and have no doubt that the timeliness and quality of the rescue were factors that allowed my recovery, but I also realize that a rescue alone cannot predict the path of recovery: be it a soldier on the field of battle, a young mother tripping down the stairs, or an athlete in an accident on the way to the game. When brain injury occurs every survivor begins a long journey. There is no way to prepare for this journey before it happens, but once it begins we can better understand it by listening to and sharing stories of recovery.

My recovery has been a gift - whether that gift comes from God or circumstance is inconsequential: I have been given the opportunity to witness and experience a full journey of recovery and to use my training and talent to better understand and share this story.

> **"**
> **A rescue alone cannot predict the path of recovery.**
> **"**

Meet Lethan Candlish

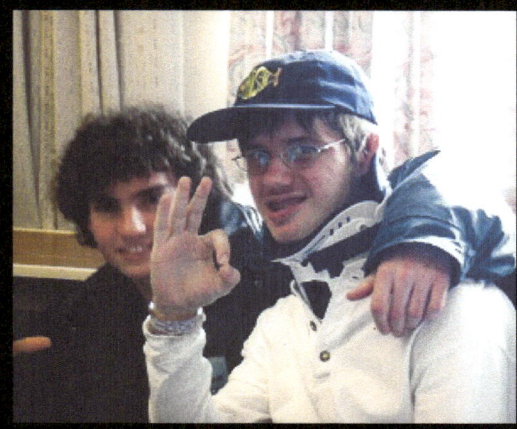

Lethan Candlish is an educator, performer, survivor, and storyteller. Having experienced TBI in 1999, Candlish was fortunate to have had a successful recovery process.

In the years that followed, as part of his MA degree focused in Storytelling, Candlish arranged the piece "Who Am I, Again" a verbal collage of stories about TBI –this piece shares events from Lethan's recovery as well as incorporating stories gathered from other survivors.

*Currently teaching English abroad, Candlish has recently returned
to reflecting upon the healing journey in his blog Who Am I, Now? Reflections on Recovery –
www. whoaminowreflections.blogspot.com.*

By terming it a "gift", I do not mean to make light of any of the tragedy in this experience - but I did survive, and by surviving believe I have gained a rare understanding of a tragic situation - this privileged understanding is what I term a gift. It is my hope that through writing and speaking publicly, other survivors and caregivers will be inspired to recognize their own tragically gained gifts. By sharing experiences, we can all help to educate the world about the realities of brain injury and recovery.

Those are some of my thoughts. For more, please visit WhoAmINowReflections.blogspot.com - there I share more of my philosophy about recovery as well an explanation of the thought process behind the performance piece "Who Am I, Again?" A verbal collage of stories about TBI. Thank you for reading and please keep in touch.

Until then, all the best and chat soon.

The key to success is action, and the essential in action is perseverance.

~Sun Yat-sen

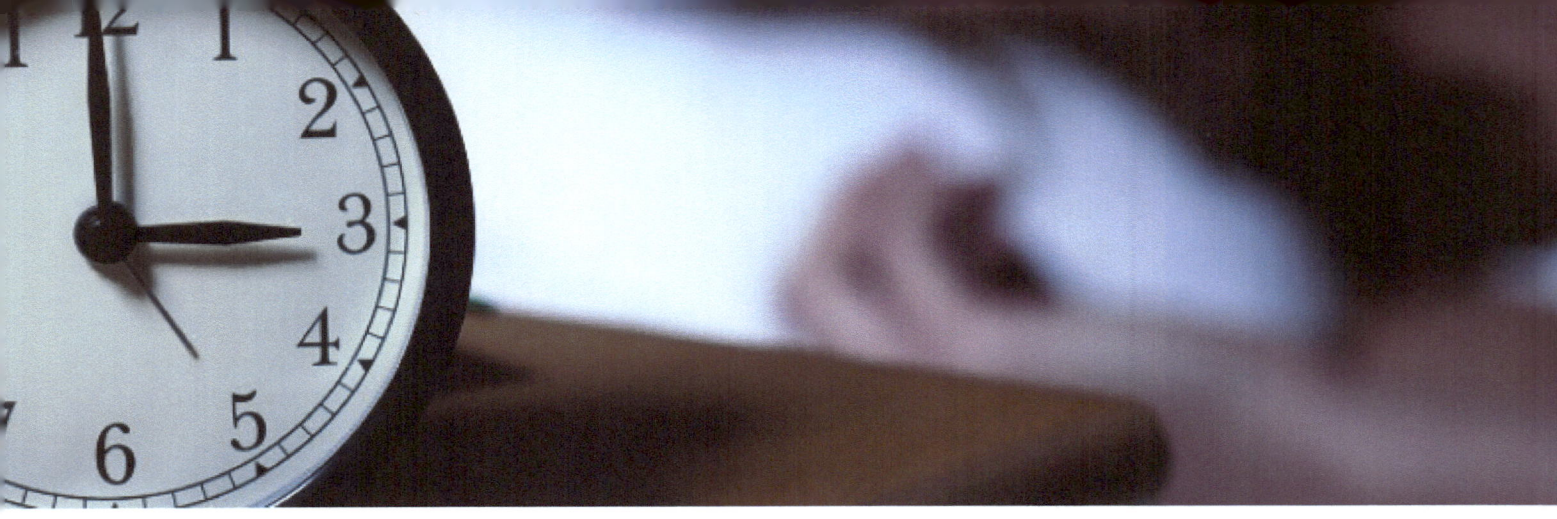

Embracing Insomnia

By Barb George

In the midst of brain trauma, one of the more prevalent issues that seem to arise is insomnia. While many people find themselves to be sleeping for inordinate amounts of time, others find themselves completely unable to get real and true restorative sleep. When this became a part of my own life nearly thirteen years ago, I dealt with it in the same manner as many… with frustration and anger. Yep. ANGER. You know the drill.

You punch the pillow… roll over, punch it again, and look at the digital clock that says some insane number such as 1:22 AM or on a good day… 3:15 AM. You get mad. You squeeze your eyes, punch the pillow (again) and lift one eyelid ten minutes later. Eventually, you give up, again looking at the clock and stumble to the coffee maker.

So, what does one do at 2 AM on a consistent basis? Creativity isn't flowing because the broken brain is taxed to the max! You can do chores if you are lucky like me and have a spouse who is hard of hearing – I can vacuum at 2 AM and he doesn't have a clue! However, one must be very careful to not do so much that when their snoozing spouse does awaken, fresh as a daisy, skipping from the bedroom, said spouse may begin to believe there are little leprechauns doing the work, rather than a very tired, brain-fried human with a busted brain. Believe me, on three hours of sleep consistently, you need people to know you really have accomplished something of value!

Reassessing this issue and after an awful lot of run-together days of anger, I made a conscious choice. I decided to 'Embrace my Insomnia.' I will be honest: it did not work well at all times. However, I continued to make the attempt. I found that if I could open one eye and see the clock and not go into anger overdrive, I might be capable of heading to the couch and dozing a bit. It didn't happen always but was possible.

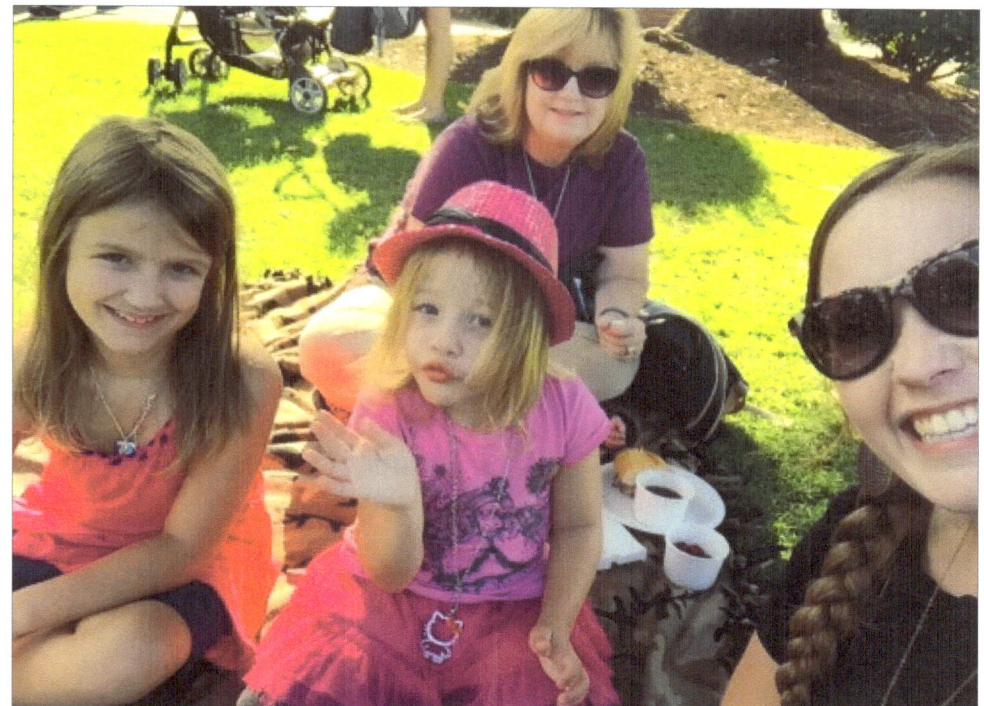

If I did not tense up my shoulders and say swear words, I might be able to sit and enjoy a TV show or read a bit (and retain more, because the anger wasn't in the way of my brain working).

If I was able to move past the frustration and into acceptance, my productivity increased! My coffee tasted better. The spouse that had such a great sleep cycle (and made me jealous) – was not on the top of my 'hit' list! I was able to have a better and fuller day!

Fast forward a number of months, and my neurologist ordered a sleep study, offering much hope for sleep apnea. I packed up my stuff, got ready for the testing after the early assessment, and settled in. At 1:45 AM I awoke. When they had me come in for the final results, I was pretty darned confident that the magic wand of a sleep machine was going to solve all my problems. My doctor picked up a box of Kleenex and handed it to me. She said, "I am so sorry, Mrs. George, you do not have sleep apnea." This was not only a shock but also sort of comical. She knew I was going to break into tears, and I did. We went over things and she gave me a few hints on 'sleep hygiene' info. I was already wearing a tracker that not only tracked my steps per day but also my sleep patterns. At the end of the visit, I drove the 50+ miles home in stunned and frustrated silence.

What to do now? Well, I have worked the entire episode into a sort of 'mini-comedy' routine that I use in our support group. It helps to laugh, but functioning on three hours of sleep each night for months on end is not productive and I can get cranky.

Since that visit, these are the things I have tried:

Benadryl: It can help, but research shows it expedites dementia. I am already on the fast track for that, due to brain trauma and family history, so I limit my use.

Prescription sleeping medications: I'm not comfortable taking them. I have memory issues and have taken more than I realized, by accident.

Essential oils: I love them. If I remember, they do help some.

Sleep Hygiene: This just sounds silly to me, but it does make sense. I know that late-night use of the phone or computer will certainly affect me. The backlighting is very bad for good sleep.

Meet Barb George

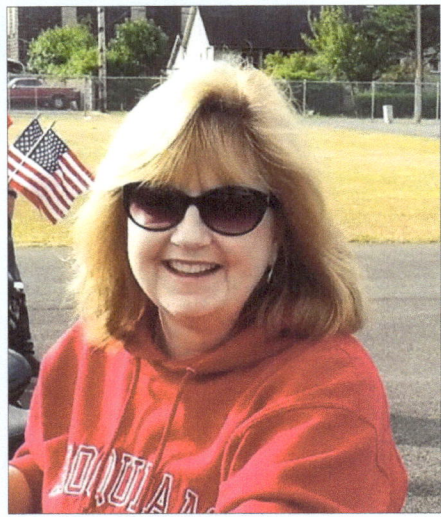

In late July of 2004, Barb was head-butted by a retired race horse, at her small hobby farm in Washington State.

Due to the rural area where she lives and the work demands of her traveling consultant husband, very little traditional therapy was available. So, working through the animals (no more horses, we changed to llamas) she was able to build up her stamina and coping skills.

After several years, through happenstance and camping trips to the ocean, it was realized that a more coastal community would be of benefit for her barometric pressure headaches. So, with health in mind, they found a smaller, more manageable, home on the coast of Washington, where they have embraced their community and life.
Barb facilitates the Grays Harbor Brain Injury Support Group and advocates for survivors and their families daily.
Barb and her husband Jim, have four adult children, and six amazing grandchildren.

TV: Don't go there, doctors. What is one to do in the dark and not look at a screen, but be bored to death for hours? My DVR has kept (some of) my sanity, but the docs do say TV is a no-no.

White noise: YES! I have used a white noise machine for 30+ years - even longer than my brain injury has been in place. I love the ocean sounds!

CBD oil and Edibles: Tried them. I am a short woman who fights her weight. Eating cookies late at night is nice, but not good in the long run for me. The CBD oil was fine - expensive - and gave me maybe 30-45 minutes of added sleep, but left me with an undesirable taste in my mouth.

Melatonin pills: They never worked that well for me.

Melatonin drops: Drops are placed under the tongue between 45-60 minutes before you hope to sleep. They relax you and help you to doze. So far, they have given me between one-to-nearly two hours of additional sleep. The difference between three and five hours of sleep is huge.

Could they be my miracle? Will Barb sleep eight hours, for the first time in thirteen years? Will Barb find peace and will her spouse no longer know by one look that she is a cranky witch at 7 AM? Is the saga over? Probably not. Will I continue on my search for sleep? Yes! One thing I know for sure is I can be angry with the clock and be cranky all day, or I can 'Embrace the Insomnia', and find a pathway to solutions and a life of enjoyment. Not perfection, but at least useful.

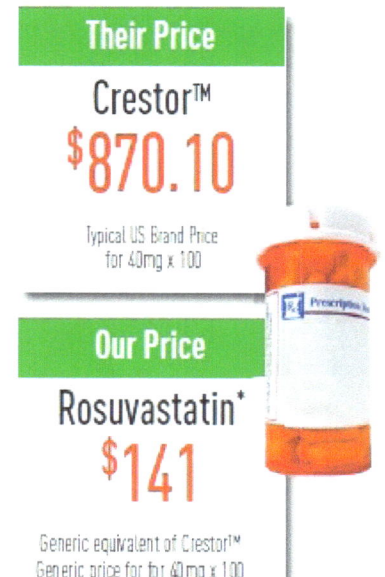 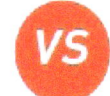 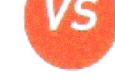
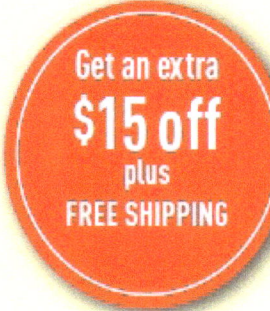
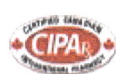 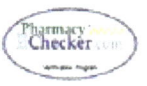 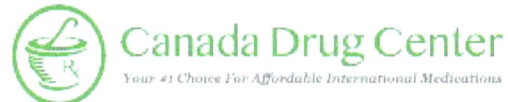

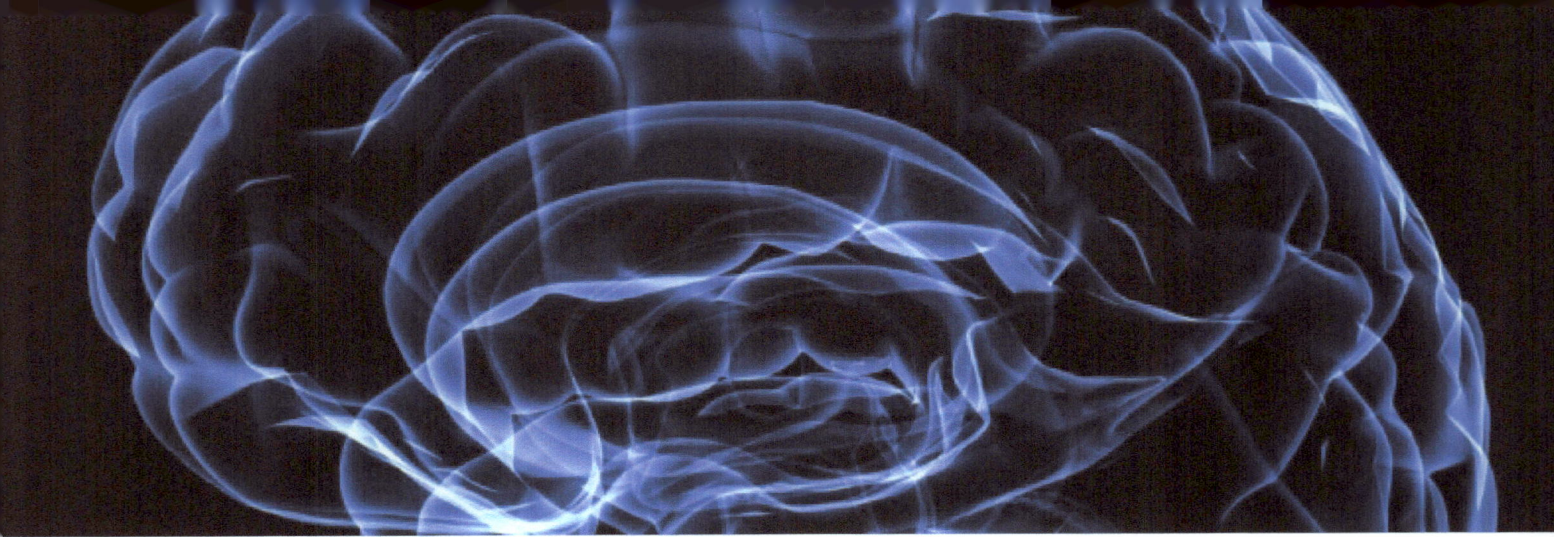

The Day I Broke My Brain

By Darron Eastwell

I have always loved mountain biking. There is something indescribably wonderful about being out on the trails. Fully immersed in nature you never know what you are going to see, and what you'll experience. Every ride is a completely unique experience.

In late May of 2015, I planned on a day of mountain bike riding at Tewantin National Park. Located on the Sunshine Coast in Queensland, Australia, Tewantin is a mountain biker's dream. The terrain is varied, with some very aggressive climbs.

It was a perfect day for riding. But, unfortunately, fate had other plans for me that day.

My GPS speedometer indicated that I had been riding for a couple of hours. As I have no memories from that day, I can only rely on the data. My pace was slow and easy as I rode. The hills were steep and I was enjoying my ride. The speedometer data show an abrupt jump in my speed up to almost 60km per hour (almost 40 MPH). It was clear that I had entered into a steep downhill descent.

This was to be the last cycling descent of my past life.

The day that started so sunny and full of bright promise ended abruptly when I crashed my mountain bike and sustained a traumatic brain injury.

Little did I know that my life, and the lives of those who love me, would be drastically changed forever. The type of brain injury that I sustained is called Diffuse Axonal Injury. I spent the next seven days in a medically induced coma. My injuries included a fractured skull, a wedge fracture to my T7 vertebrae, and a fracture to my neck.

Post Traumatic Amnesia affected my memory to the point of having no memory of that fateful day, with the memory of my mountain biking accident forever erased from my brain. I cannot tell you where it happened, how it happened, the pain I was in, the ambulance ride to ICU or being admitted to three different hospitals over the two months that followed.

About the only memory I have been able to retain was of being discharged from the hospital. I had met the recovery expectations of the medical staff, so I was allowed to leave to continue my rehab and recovery on an outpatient basis.

I was advised by my occupational therapist that to help assist with improving my memory, speech and fine motor skills, I should start to write a daily journal of what happened, and what I had done or was supposed to have done during the day. To this day, I can't remember when I started writing my journal however, very slowly the words started coming out. I did the best I could to put them down on paper.

My handwriting was adversely affected by my brain injury. Before my injury, I had very neat handwriting and could write very quickly and legibly.

After my injury, my writing was the complete opposite. It was messy with numerous spelling mistakes. Just like my new speech challenges, it was not flowing easily or naturally. Using a computer brought no relief as I had forgotten how to use it and was suddenly unfamiliar with the keyboard

I persisted with my new chicken-scratch handwriting, trying my best to remember and write down my thoughts. I don't know how long I had been writing my journal, though I think it was approximately twelve months before I could sense some improvement with my writing, language, speech, and concentration. My memory and neuro-fatigue were still the biggest challenges I faced. It was at that point that I read several books about TBI survival and recovery.

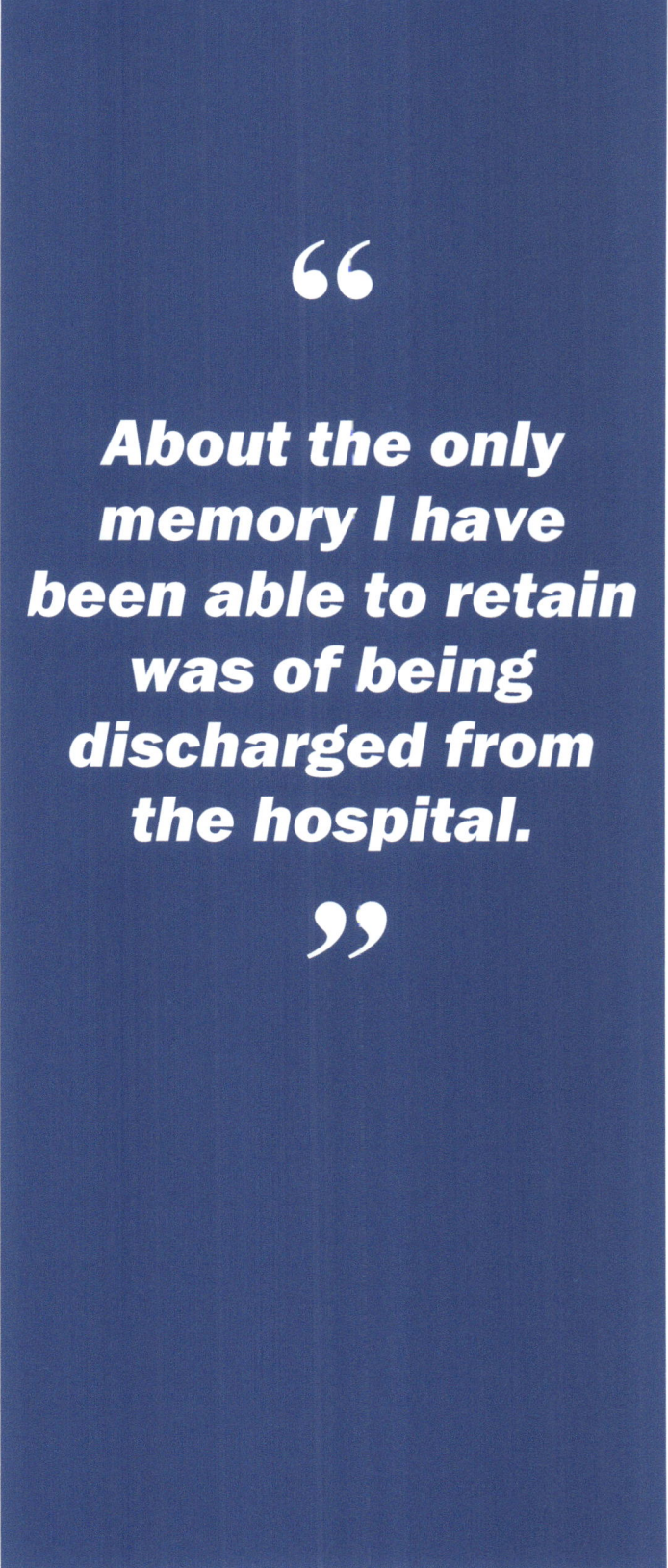

" About the only memory I have been able to retain was of being discharged from the hospital. "

Prior to my injury, I had never heard or read about TBI.

I said to myself, "Darron you need to write a book about your own TBI story as it will help you, but more importantly, it could help other TBI survivors and their families that are going through what you have gone through."

This is when my book, *The Day I Broke My Brain,* started on paper.

I re-read my journal notes as often as I could because I couldn't always remember what I had written. Diligently, I would pen chapter suggestions and topics to write about. It took me almost a year of writing. Writing a book was entirely new to me as I had never set out to do anything like it before. Like so much of life after brain injury, it was unchartered territory for me.

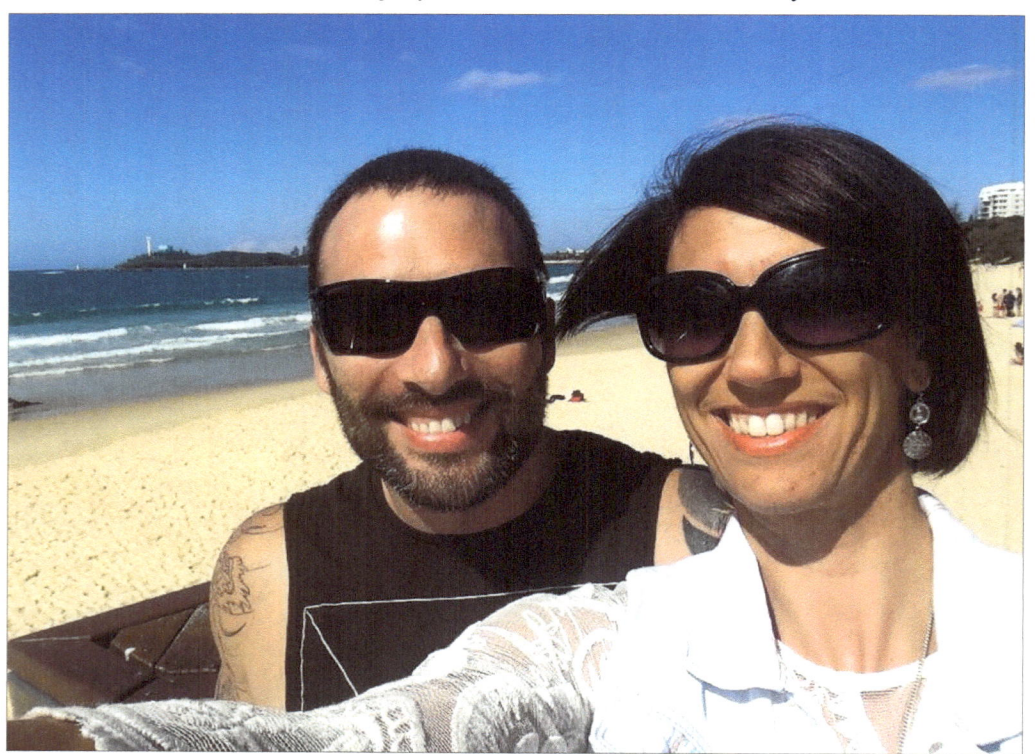

At this point in time, my story was entirely handwritten. I knew that to get the book project started, I needed to be able to email what I had written. My next step was to type up my scribbled handwritten notes so that I would have a readable format. I set myself up to type a few pages on a daily basis. I set myself a goal to have it completed within a month's time.

The typing was very much a form of rehab and mental stimulation at the same time. Though the overall process was very rewarding, after a couple of long days of typing I suffered from bad neuro-fatigue. It knocked me out for days, I was so mentally exhausted. This happened several times as I worked my way through the typing out of my book. I took the required breaks to help myself recover, and then I would start again. I was determined to finish.

A full month later, I completed typing the first draft of my upcoming book. The Day I Broke My Brain was born!

I was feeling really proud of myself, given what I had already been through. While writing my book, I was still recovering from my brain injury and all the TBI difficulties it brings to me on a daily basis. Writing my book is one of the most satisfying things that I ever have done in my life.

Meet Darron Eastwell

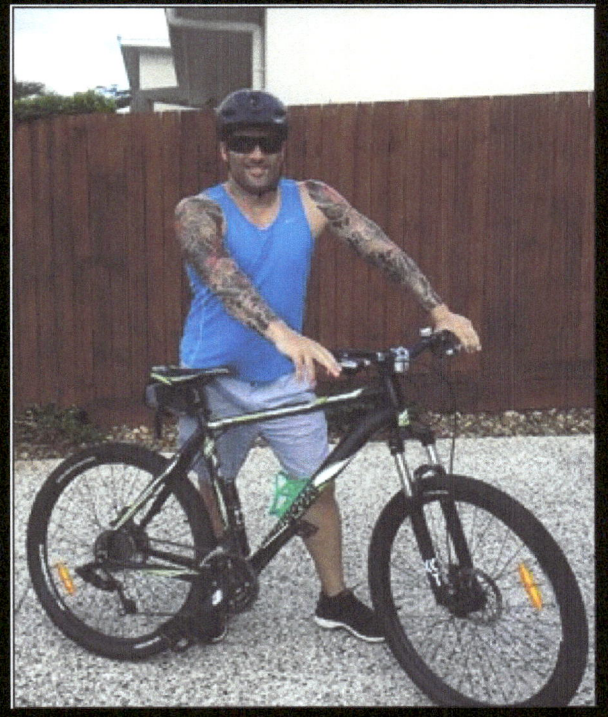

Darron Eastwell is a brain injury survivor from Queensland, Australia.

The survivor of a 2015 mountain biking accident, Darron has emerged with a strong desire to serve those within the brain injury community.

His first title, "The Day I Broke My Brain," is scheduled for release on Amazon in June of 2017.

Darron and his wife Bianca share their love for their two children and have embraced their new life together.

I still can't believe it really. I am actually going to have a book about my own TBI story. This is so exciting. The main purpose of writing my TBI story is to provide help to other TBI survivors and their families. My hope is that my new book may provide them with hope, motivation, and inspiration to keep positive and push themselves during their own recovery process. Readers may try something I did during my own recovery that assisted me, as it could help with their own recovery.

I have a framed quote in my lounge room. It was something I looked at regularly and read on a weekly basis.

It reads as follows…

"Sometimes the best thing you can do is not think, not wonder, not imagine, just breathe and have faith that everything will work out for the best."

I have used this statement as a kind of mantra to help me to live in the moment and not look too far ahead during my recovery. I still do it to this day.

I believe that everything in life happens for a reason. I often say to myself that I survived my TBI so that my experience can help others.

At this time, I am almost two years out from my accident, an accident that gave me life membership as a brain injury survivor. My recovery is still improving and today I love my life.

I hope to never forget that I am one of the lucky ones.

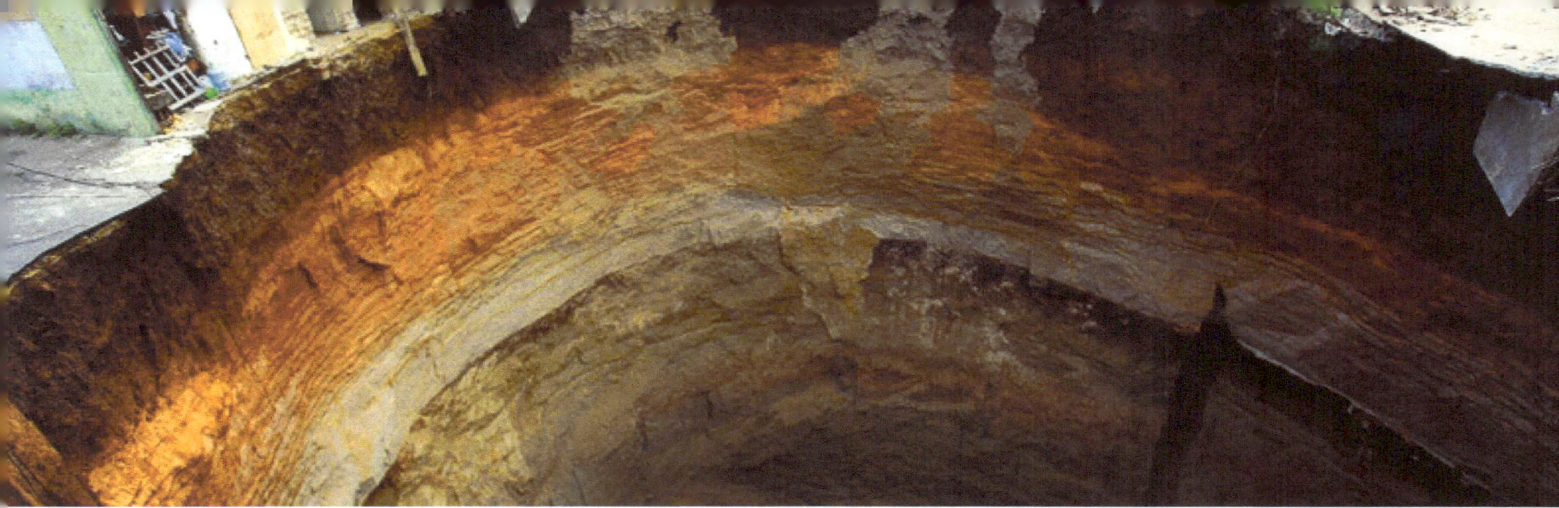

The Sinkhole
By Ralph Poland

Since I had my strokes, I have been trying to find words to offer insight for those who have not suffered any type of brain injury. Then, one night last month while trying to get back to sleep, the following came to mind.

Equating a brain injury to personally experiencing a sinkhole.

Imagine yourself strolling along in your life journey while setting your sights on your present plans and looking towards the horizon with goals, aspirations, and ambitions, in your foreseeable future.

When, in a flash, the ground beneath your feet abruptly drops with you going down with it. As you are falling, you're realizing that you were on top of what has suddenly turned into a very large sinkhole. Once the dust settles, you struggle to dig yourself out of the very dense mud, enough to hopelessly stand at the bottom within a **Very Dark, Deep, Isolated** yet **Lonely** and **Unstable Sinkhole**. At some point, you notice other **Various Elements** of your former life had also come crashing down with you but, those elements are now scattered in unrepairable pieces, partially buried nearby or even haphazardly strewn all around you.

At that point, you begin to find yourself experiencing many stages of feelings, such as - **Anger** - **Bitterness - Depression, - Fear - Frustration** - and, of being **Overwhelmed**.

Then, as you are noticing more and more aspects of your former life still caving in around you, it seems like anything left of your former life is still haphazardly hanging just overhead. You try to grab each of them in desperate hopes to climb your way up and out (back to your normal life) but, sadly, you're finding that what you grabbed onto also comes crashing down around you.

Meanwhile, your friends and family are hopelessly looking on while experiencing **Bewilderment**, and unable to offer you any kind of **Help/Hope** that may assist you in finding your own way, as you start to search for ways to begin to climb back out of that **Horrible Sinkhole** you are experiencing, in an attempt to resume your former life.

Over time, one by one, strangers slowly appear dropping **Ropes*** down to you, as a form of Aid to help you to climb out. Some ropes only help you to a certain extent, while other ropes help a great deal more. Still, you find it very difficult to gain a footing to climb up further. But eventually, many of those strangers (these being Therapists) offer you some strategies that help you to slowly begin to climb up.

~This is just an illustration of what many Brain Injury survivors are experiencing right after suffering any type of Acquired Brain Injury. ~

Finally, months or years later, most of us can struggle our way up enough to eventually reach the top. However, even then, it remains a challenging struggle to climb on out and find stable enough ground to stand on, only to discover that even that bit of ground is shifting **Daily**, from then on.

*Those of you who are our Doctors - Nurses - CNAs – Dietitians - Therapists and other Members of our Medical Team are the ones working to rescue us, by dropping the ropes down to us. Due to this, "Thank you" is not nearly enough to express our gratitude.

Meet Ralph Poland

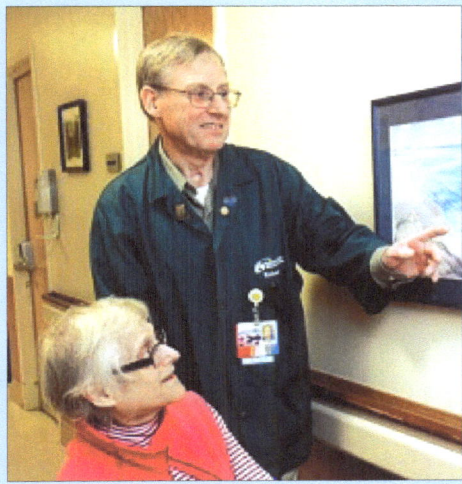

Since re-inventing himself the past seven years, Ralph now works part time at a local Wal-Mart. He also volunteers at a local hospital. His real passion is volunteering at the Rehab where he recovered. There, he shares his story with patients, offering them hope and inspiration.

Ralph also serves on the BIA-MAINE Chapter, as well as on CMMC's Patient Advisory Council. He continues to offer insight from a brain injured survivor's perspective to support groups, Neuro OT students at UNE, and staff members at CMMC.

Live life to the fullest, and focus on the positive.

~Matt Cameron

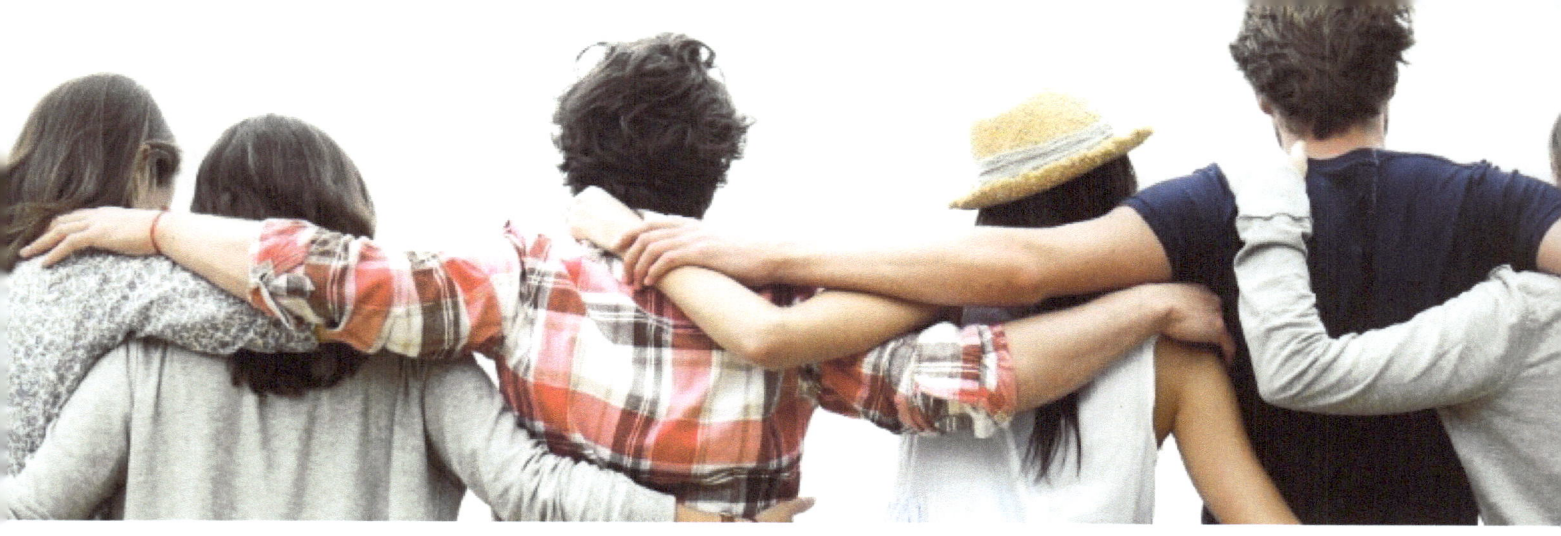

To Support Group or Not

By Donna O'Donnell Figurski

These days, there are support groups for almost everything. Probably the most well-known group is "AA" (Alcoholics Anonymous). There are groups for eating disorders, domestic abuse, mental health, physical health problems, such as cancer and diabetes, groups to enhance relationships, and many others. If there is a problem, there is probably a group for folks to join. Groups for supporting brain-injury survivors and their caregivers, family members, and friends are cropping up everywhere. This is relatively new since little was known about the seriousness of brain injury until rather recently. When the troops began to come home from the Iraq war with serious brain injuries, people started to notice. Then when the deaths and illnesses of so many former NFL players came to light - starting with Dr. Omalu's finding of chronic traumatic encephalopathy (CTE) in the brain of Pittsburgh Steeler Mike Webster during an autopsy in 2002 - more people took notice.

Two things you might consider when searching for a support group are the location (Is it within reach? Will you easily be able to get there?) and size (Is it large enough or small enough for you? Too large – you may get lost and not have any of your needs met. Too small – there may not be enough information to share, but it may be easier to connect with folks with the same interests). You will need to comfort-fit your support group to your needs. If you are unable to join an in-person support group, don't fret. There are many support groups on social media.

My husband's brain injury happened in January of 2005. As his caregiver, I went it alone … for years and years. I wasn't aware of the multitude of people who had a brain injury. I was ignorant that there were millions of caregivers like me, and I certainly never realized that there were support groups for caregivers. It wasn't until three years ago that I stumbled onto the support groups on Facebook. I joined many of them, and I have made many good friends there - both virtual (some from across the world) and the ones nearer, some of whom I met in person to share a coffee or a lunch together.

There are virtual groups for caregivers. (One is just for spouses or partners of survivors.) There are groups for both survivors and caregivers together. There are groups for traumatic brain injury survivors; for acquired brain injury survivors; or, for survivors with ataxia, multiple sclerosis, or stroke.

Some of the benefits of support groups are that folks are more apt to understand what you are going through. Since they share similar issues, they are able to offer emotional support, suggest advice, or provide tips that worked for them. There is a veritable smorgasbord of ideas out there in cyber world. If you are looking for an online group to hold your hand, hear you vent, or answer your questions, I promise you will find it.

Support groups are usually, but not always, beneficial. When my husband, David, had his brain injury in 2005, I had little knowledge of support groups. We went to a local group a few times, but David didn't find it helpful. In fact, for him, so early in his journey, it was not at all beneficial. He found it difficult to identify with the other survivors of brain injury.

Though David was in poor shape physically and was unable to do much for himself, he still felt that his mental health condition was better than that of the others in the group. Being in the group brought David down and left him with little hope. He asked that we not go back, and I agreed. But, unlike this example, many people rely on support groups.

Because our earth supports more than twenty-four different time zones, there is always someone available to talk with 24/7. That is one of the major advantages of belonging to support groups on social media, and I am so grateful that I stumbled onto them. I finally knew that David and I weren't alone. Just in the United States, there are more than five million people living with brain injury. Can you imagine the number if you counted up all of the survivors of brain injury around the world? Astronomical!

If you are not yet convinced that support groups can be helpful for you, here are a few more reasons: They empower you. They put you in the driver's seat to take control of what is happening in your life by helping you to find answers. You immediately become a member of a like-minded group of people who accept you, understand you, and are not judgmental. So, if you feel a support-group would be beneficial to you, by all means, find one. They can be wonderful!

So, how do you find a support group to comfort-fit your needs? If you choose to be a part of an in-person support group, ask your primary-care provider, your neurologist, a social worker, or your church minister to recommend any groups near you. You may also contact the Brain Injury Association of America (BIAUSA.org) and locate your local chapter for your state to find a support group near you.

But, if you prefer the comfort of your home (as I do) and you have nimble fingers, open up your computer and find a Facebook group. There are more than thirty to join. I know - because I am a member of at least thirty. I only wish that I had known about the social media support groups when David had his brain injury over eleven years ago. With a support group, you are never alone.

Meet Donna O'Donnell Figurski

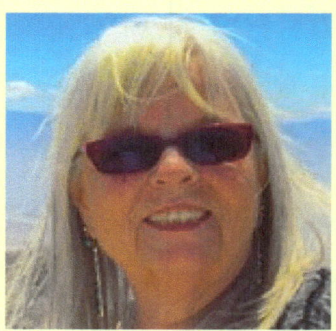

Donna O'Donnell Figurski is a wife, mother, and granny. She is a teacher, playwright, actor, director, writer, picture-book reviewer.

On January 13, 2005, Donna became the caregiver for her husband and best friend, David. Donna had never heard of "TBI" before David's cerebellar hemorrhage.

Donna spends each day writing a blog, called "Surviving Traumatic Brain Injury," and preparing for her radio show, "Another Fork in the Road," on the Brain Injury Radio Network.

"How long is recovery?" squeaked Piglet.

"For most people, it's lifelong," said Pooh.

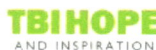

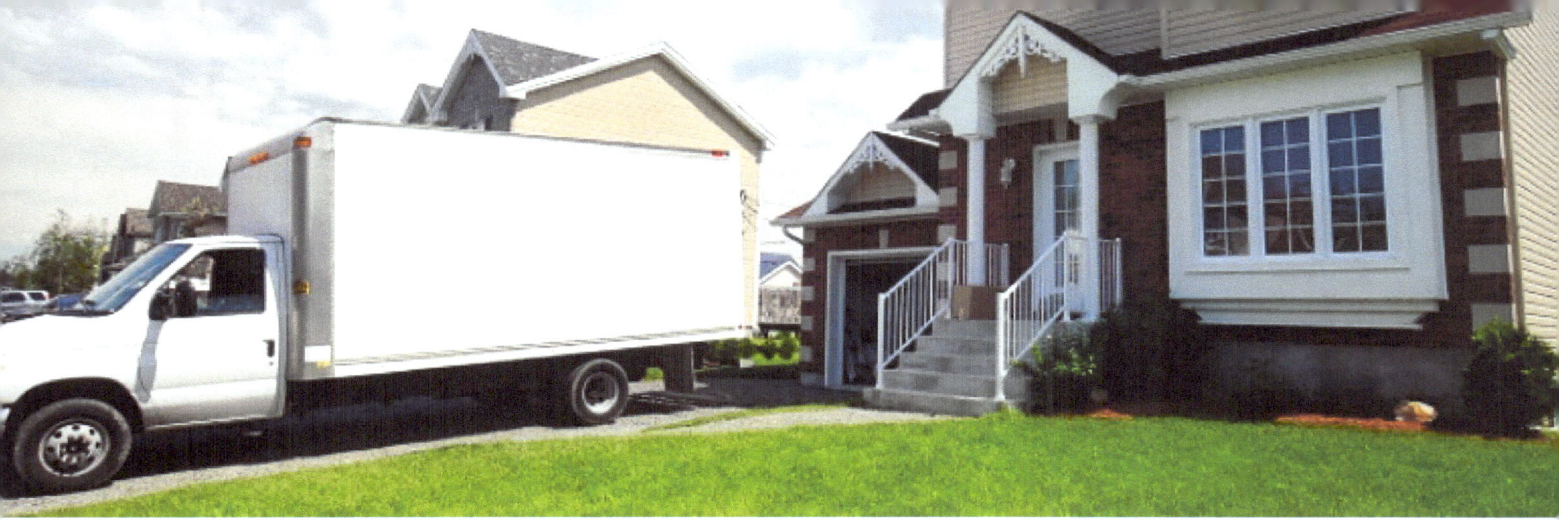

My New Start

By Natalie Griffith

In July of 2016, my ex-husband told me he was moving with my kids, to another state - Texas; he had been struggling to raise our four kids by himself since my TBI, seven years prior. First and foremost, he has done an amazing job raising our growing children who are 18, 16, 14, & 10½ and I couldn't be more grateful! Am I fully recovered? Lol, I think we all keep recovering forever after a brain injury and we achieve little milestones for the rest of our lives!

When he told me about his decision, I didn't know what to think. I was working in a brand new hotel, greeting guests as they picked out their breakfast items and seated themselves. I would say hi and check on them, then pick up dirty empty plates, and cleaned everything afterward so it looked presentable. Wow, I loved it! I found that I could remember what I was doing if I walked away, and multitask without feeling overwhelmed. It took about 1-1½ months for the rhythm to sink in.

Since my accident, I've found that I need consistency, rhythm, and accuracy. I can handle things and make due if it's not that way, but it's just slower to fully think about what needs to be done because my brain works differently since my injury. During my breakfast shifts, I got to know some of the long-term guests. One of the guests was visiting California with her family because they loved the beach and they were moving - from Texas!

I mentioned that my children were moving and her comment to me, which I believe was ordained by God, was, "In my opinion, isn't it better for your recovery to be near your children?" She had been staying at the hotel for a long while and she knew my Second Chance story, and how my kids, along with God, had been the focal point of my recovery.

I went home from work wondering, thinking, and praying, and the next morning, I gave my two-week notice - I was moving! Born and raised in California, I am a beach girl (going to the beach lying in the sun, helped my brain heal). My youngest sister lived in Texas with her family so I would know someone and have support there! I made the decision to move before the transfer to another hotel went through. I had struggled so much, living in different rooms in California, because it was so expensive. I was trying to get back on my feet and it was very hard to find a job I could handle as I recovered. I have never lived in my own place. I went from my parents' home to marriage, then with a roommate because of my separation, and then moved from room to room because I didn't have much money or a stable job. It was a crazy idea to move as I didn't have much holding me in California, except family and close church

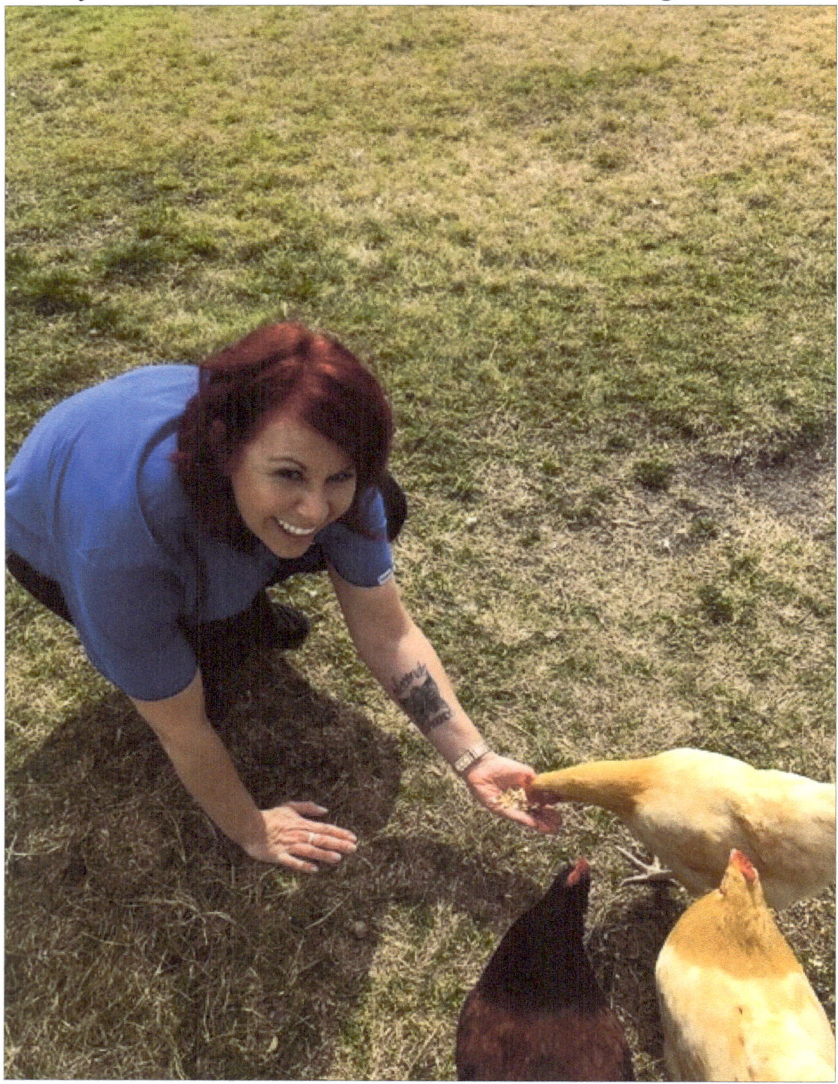

friends. My faith has been in God and I believe I was saved for a purpose; for He has a plan, and maybe that would be in Texas?

About a week after I gave my notice, my transfer went through so I could start at another Hilton hotel in Austin Texas, doing roughly the same thing: Breakfasts, Banquets, Serving in their restaurant, and Room Service. Before my TBI, I was a waitress. I'm a people person so I thoroughly enjoyed what I did. I hadn't put much thought into moving to another state and I hardly had belongings because of living in the different rooms (five different rooms in six years.) I thought it would be easy to drive by myself; I had just about died and I COULD DO ANYTHING!

My mom was not okay with my decision and rearranged her schedule to drive with me (she had been planning on going the week after to visit my sister, her family, and kids anyway). We did the nineteen-hour drive in three days, staying at hotels in different states. What a beautiful drive!

Everything I had (not much) was piled in plastic bins which were packed in my Kia Sorrento. The drive from California to Arizona, to New Mexico, then to Hutto, Texas, was a pure green beauty: beautifully shaped rocks, light beige/brown color of the dirt on the hills with some green - simply gorgeous. You may have seen ugly brown dirt in a long, hot drive, but all I could see was the beauty of the creation of God! Thanks to my TBI, all I see is pure beauty in everything.

We arrived at my sister's home in Hutto, Texas on a Friday and when we got there I had no place to go, so I camped at my sister's home with my mom that evening. The next morning, she and I looked at a few different apartments in my price range, close to where my ex-husband and kids were living. I still had to be careful financially because my new job in Texas didn't pay as much as my old job in California.

The apartment I chose had "Summer" as part of the name, so at least it gave me a hint of California, which made me feel better. My ex-husband rented a house and offered to let me stay with them (sleeping in my youngest daughter's bunkbed) until my apartment was ready; I am grateful for such kindness.

Six months into living in this new state, I'm on my third job: caregiving, which is amazing because I have such heart, such love, and compassion for the old and disabled. The clients I have are in their seventies.

I am learning about myself and what I can do through helping them, which is a gift from God! Although I still have minor memory issues, I inspire myself to keep going, keep trying and mostly to NOT GIVE UP. God is good!

Do not let your grand ambitions stand in the way of small but meaningful accomplishments.
~Bryant H. McGill

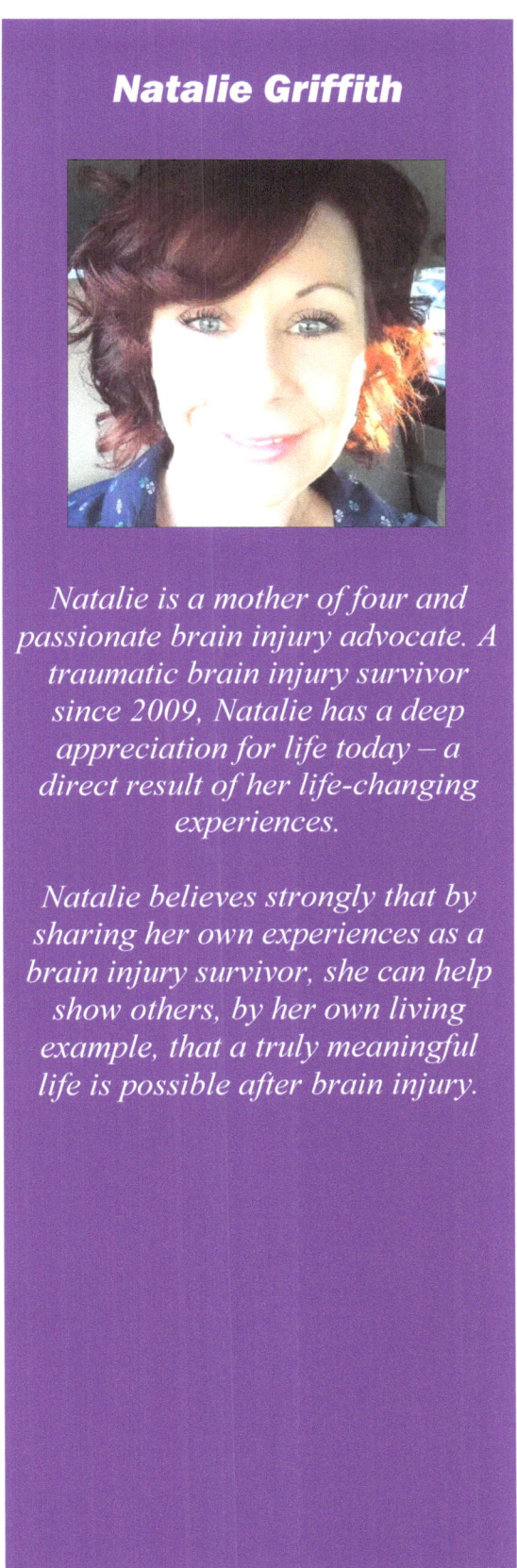

Natalie Griffith

Natalie is a mother of four and passionate brain injury advocate. A traumatic brain injury survivor since 2009, Natalie has a deep appreciation for life today – a direct result of her life-changing experiences.

Natalie believes strongly that by sharing her own experiences as a brain injury survivor, she can help show others, by her own living example, that a truly meaningful life is possible after brain injury.

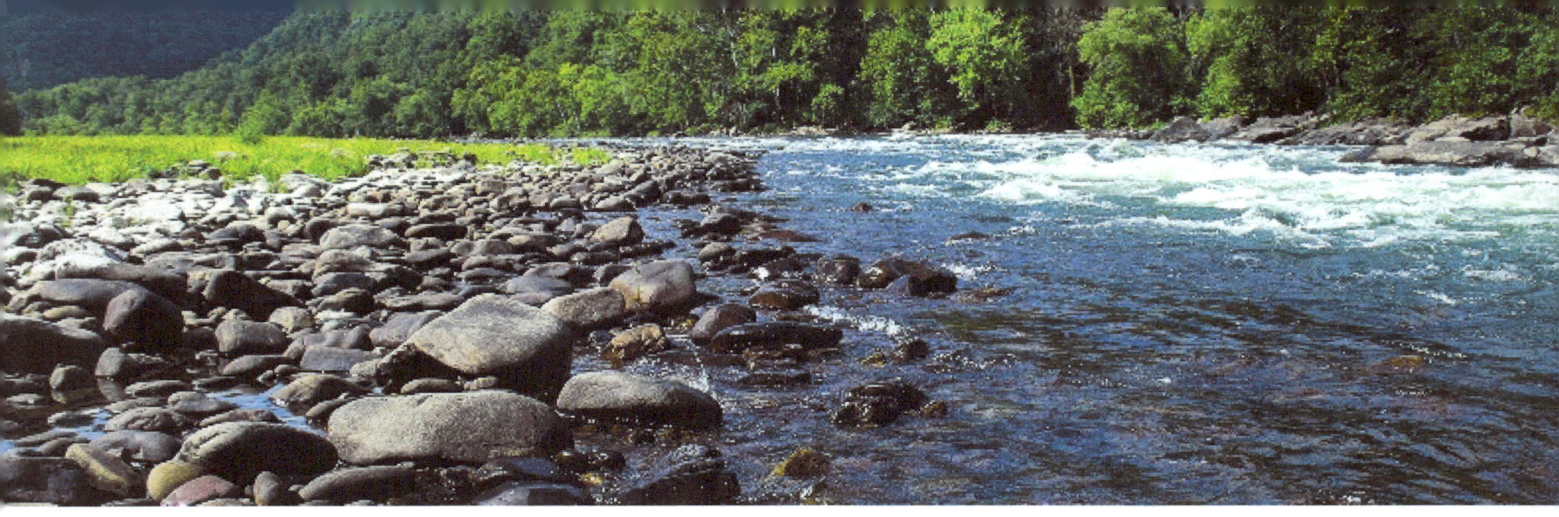

Acknowledge the Impact

By Nicole Bingaman

I have a hobby of sorts that has helped me profoundly as I journey with my son through his recovery from brain injury, and my own journey of what I have recently come to acknowledge as post-traumatic stress disorder.

The first sign of PTSD happened a few years ago when the sounds of a life-flight helicopter cut through my being as if it were a literal knife, touching my skin. I'm referring to the sound of the whooshing of the helicopter blades. Each whoosh represented a previously unfelt level of fear and anguish. It was not as if I wanted to duck, but instead, needed to run and hide from what the noise represented, loss of control, and the potential loss of life.

I recently needed to undergo some medical tests. As the various procedures started, I recognized a level of fear not previously present in me. On that particular day, I wore socks that depicted a little girl riding her bike, with blonde pigtails, and the words, "Hell raiser" printed across the top. The socks served as a personal reminder, "You got this."

Once the needle was inserted with the camera to guide the imaging, tears began to fall. There happened to be a fellow yoga classmate's son on the team, who recognized me. I confided in him that I felt incredibly vulnerable and frightened. As the team began talking with me, I told them I wore the wrong socks. I should have worn socks with a cat, whose hair was standing on its head, with the word, "YIKES!"

Over the next few hours, there were more needles and tests, none of which were invasive or profoundly awful, but my heart and head pounded with an intense anxiety that I was not going to be okay. The people around me entered into a new kind of mode. They held my hand, spoke firm but soothing words, and reminded me that to get through the entire ordeal, I was going to have to endure some pain.

As the MRI machine clamored loudly in my ears, one of the technicians stayed at my feet for the entire hour, rubbing my toes, whispering reassuring words whenever I wiggled them, and reminding me that I was not alone.

I thought a lot about my son and the many surgeries and tests he has undergone. I thought about the hundreds of staples that were not only removed from his head, but also forced inside of his soft skin. I thought about my dear friend and her lengthy struggle with breast cancer and all that she's endured, and I told myself, "You've got to toughen up. This is simple and you are strong." But I felt violently afraid. Real fear assaulted me and in those moments, I realized that the aftermath of my son's brain injury continued to show up in unexpected ways.

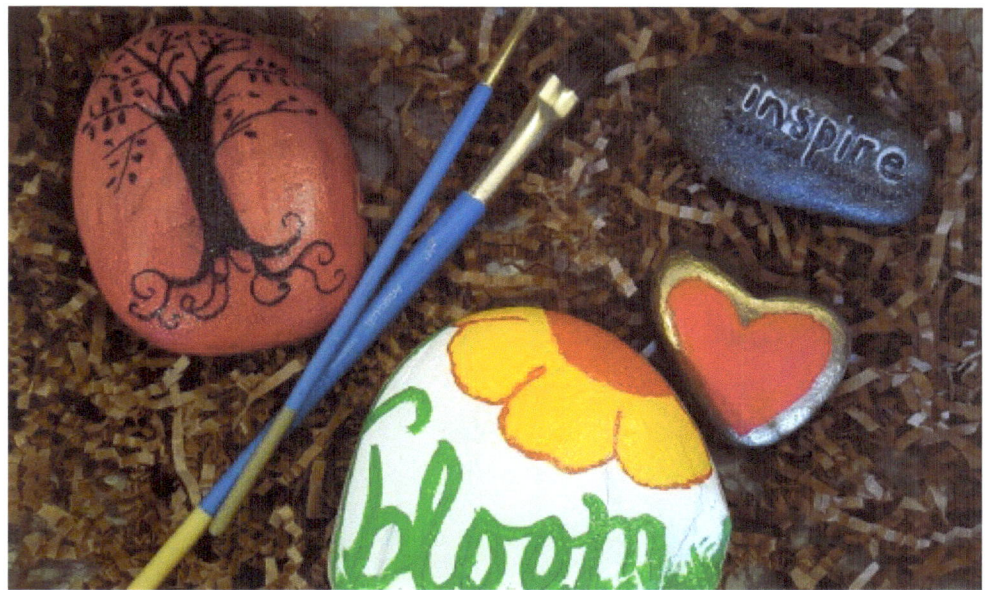

The problem is, life is going to go on. In moving forward, more heartache, pain and uncomfortable scenarios are bound to occur. In order to stay the course with my survivor, I have to work on acquiring another skillset, which in this case meant acknowledging the unseen impact of the trauma I've witnessed.

Later that night I thought about all that I felt, and wondered why it had reared its ugly head on this day.

For hours, as I sat in the waiting areas, or in various rooms of the hospital there was a screen playing in a teeny-tiny corner of my mind. On the screen were clips from the days in the intensive care unit, the muffled cries of people saying their final goodbyes to a loved one, the endless beeps and alarms, and sometimes the frantic race of nurses and doctors, as they attempted to save a life.

My mind replayed visions of myself, in a waiting room, with a threadbare blanket, a makeshift pillow and a cold that reached into my bones, as I drifted in and out, pondering these things… "How did my son get here?" "Would I say goodbye to him, as I had my stepbrother and my sister?"

Trauma replayed, over and over again. Death seemed to be staring me down.

One of the harshest realities that brain injury has taught me is that on this earth, we will experience great joy, which may be accompanied by an even greater sorrow.

People speak of karma, and reaping what you sow. Figuring out what that means as you lie across your son's legs, begging God for him to stay, is hard. It is like a slap in the face to your spirit, over and over again, until suddenly you realize your cheeks are bleeding from the pain, but you know there's more.

Not all brain injury survivors live in a forever scenario. Depending on the level of recovery, countless survivors learn to navigate through life, embracing the concept of a whole new world. For others the injury is more profound.

There are survivors living in a nursing home, or with round the clock care. Some will never walk, speak or eat again. There are wives who will have forever lost all but their husband's shell, and fathers who will never again hear the words, "Daddy." Many TBI warriors win small battles, only to fight an ongoing war. That is the cycle of TBI life.

One of my new hobbies is painting rocks. I paint one word…hope, gratitude, or peace. I start by finding the perfect rock at the local farm and garden store, and then I choose a color for the first layer. From there I decide what I need to feel and be in the next few days, and let my brush take flight.

In creating something simple that doesn't take countless hours, or hundreds of redo's, I center myself and I see that there is something good inside of the pain. Even if it is nothing more than pretty colors on a rock reminding me of a truth I can embrace.

Our human compassion binds us the one to the other.

~Nelson Mandela

Meet Nicole Bingaman

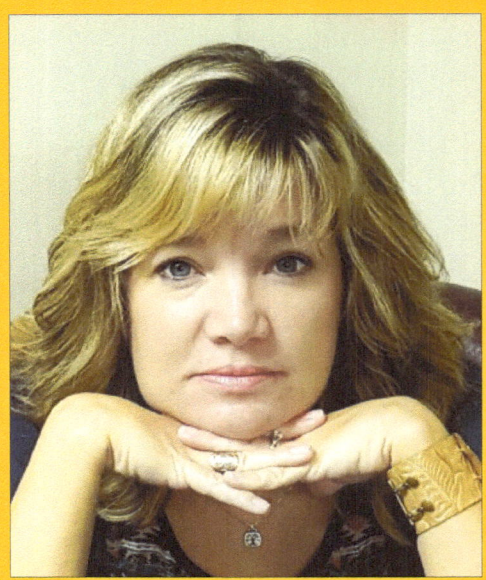

Nicole has worked in the human service field for over twenty years. Since Taylor's injury Nicole has become an advocate and spokesperson within the TBI community.

Nicole's book "Falling Away From You" was published and released in 2015. Nicole continues to share Taylor's journey on Facebook. Nicole firmly believes in the mantra that "Love Wins."

Learn more at www.nicolebingaman.com

While I wear a lot of hats these days, from husband to father, from worker to friend, I am a brain injury surivor.

Like every survivor I have ever met, I still have significant life challenges. Catch me on a "good TBI day," and you might never notice my disability. But the pendulum swings both ways. On a tough day, just getting my shoes tied can be the highlight of my day.

Fortunately, as time passes, so does the frequency of my tough days. But they still come, unasked for, and often at the most inopportune of times. It's called life on life's terms.

Last month's edition of the print version of TBI HOPE Magazine has proven to be an unparalleled success. Like many other survivors, I have light sensitivity. There are times when my monitor or tablet feels like it's boring holes in my head. Light quickly converts to pain. Again, it is what it is.

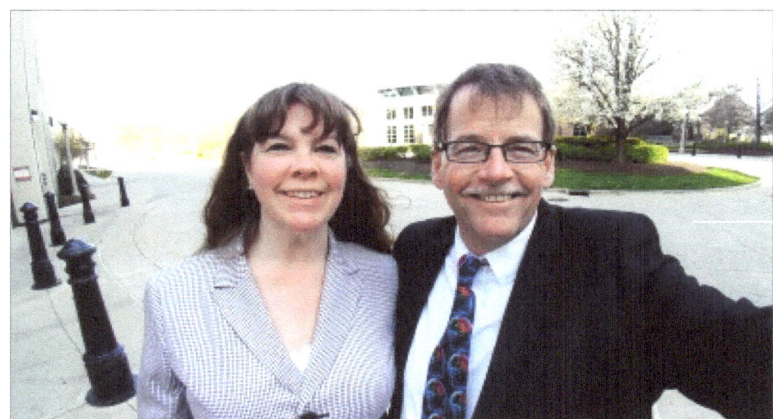

Over the last couple of years, many survivors have asked us for a print version – something to hold, to refer back to, to make notes in, and to read away from the artificial environment that comes with having only a digital publication. My wife Sarah and I spent over a year looking for a viable print partner that would work well for our readers. As we explored our options, Amazon became the clear print partner to work with.

From ultra-thick paper stock to an impeccable full-color interior print to free shipping for Prime members, it's clear that the choice we made will benefit our readers.

We have already had a number of agencies and organizations reach out to us for volume orders of the magazine. They are bringing copies in-house to hand out at support groups and to pass on to case workers for distribution to the brain injury community. If you are part of a brain injury organization and would like more information, let me know at david@tbihopeandinspiration.com

As we move forward through 2017, watch for more exciting news as we continue to evolve as a premier provider of forward-moving information and resources to those who share our fate.

~David & Sarah Grant

www.ingramcontent.com/pod-product-compliance
Lightning Source LLC
Chambersburg PA
CBHW060812290526
45792CB00005BA/1630